# THE HIRATA ZONE
# COLOURING
## AND WORKBOOK

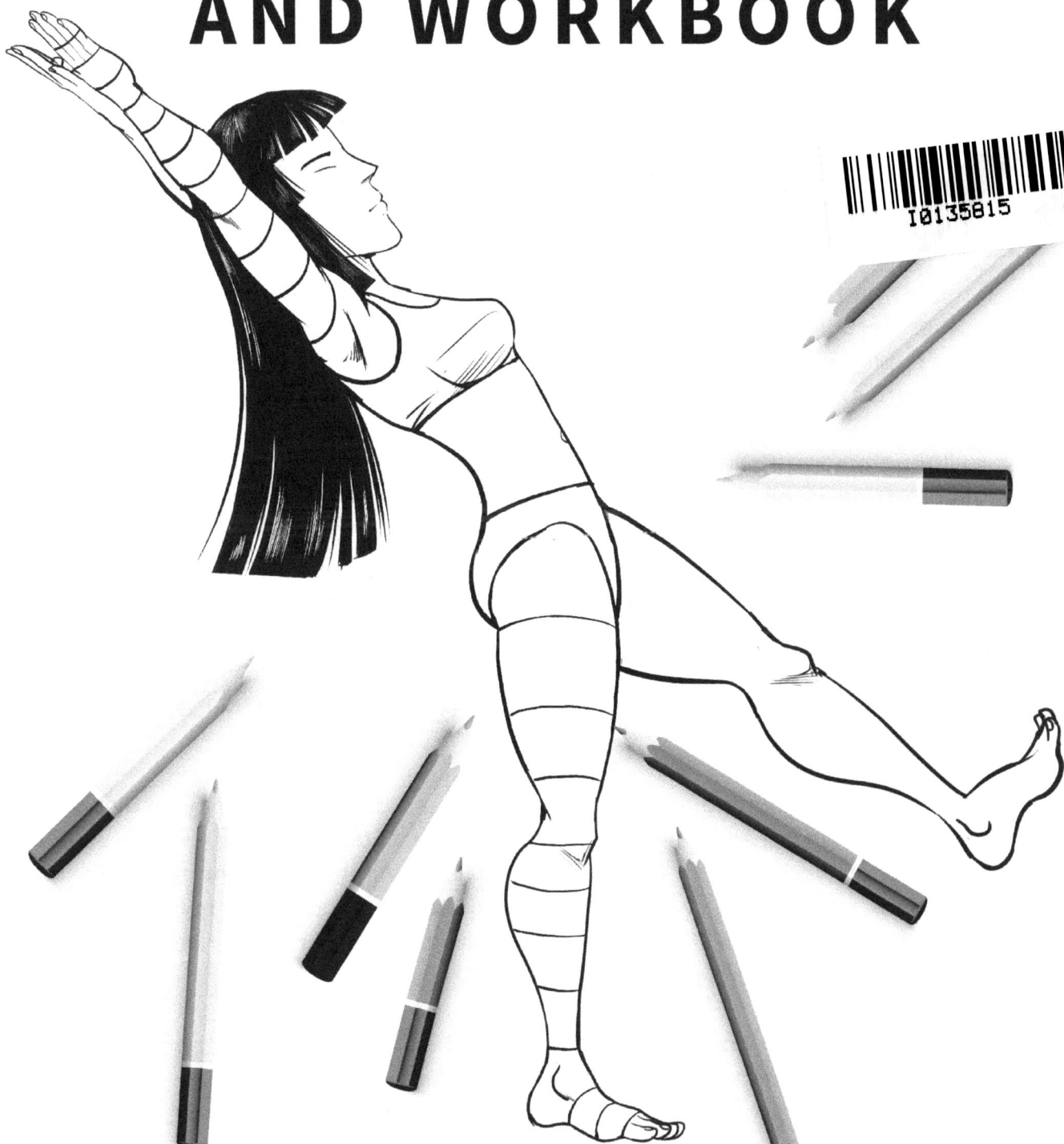

I0135815

## ORAN KIVITY

*Cover Design: Jietwong.com*

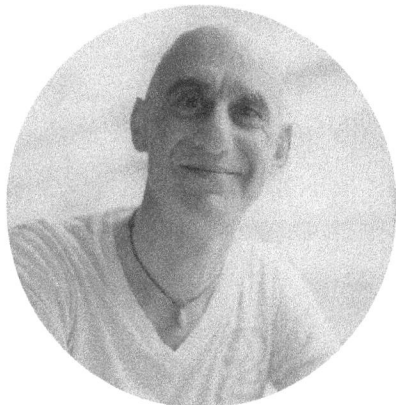

# A NOTE FROM THE AUTHOR

## WELCOME TO THIS COLOURING BOOK

When I first learned Hirata Zone Therapy, the first thing to figure out was where the zones actually were. The second thing was finding a way to memorise the zone numbering and names.

As the main book progressed, I got the idea to design a simple colouring book as a free downloadable study aid. Both in personal growth and education, we find clarity through expression. I hope that by drawing and colouring, you'll be able to memorise these locations and correlations. The free download covers Chapter 7 of the main book.

Of course, as with all my "simple" ideas, the project got bigger than first planned, and I couldn't help myself from developing more exercises and worksheets! The free download idea got superseded by the idea of a professionally printed paperback to accompany the main book. In addition to being better laid out, the paperback contains new study material. These extra worksheets and diagrams will help you get to grips with the metronome frequencies and the principles of applying Basic Hirata. If you're happy with home printing the free downloadable PDF (the link is in the main book), you can ignore this one. But if you'd like some extra information and a well-produced paperback to work through, then this is the book for you!

I hope you find it useful. Most importantly, I hope it makes your learning fun.

*Oran Kivity*

Oran Kivity
Kaohsiung, Taiwan, 2021

# INTRO CHECKLIST

WHAT YOU NEED TO DO

INSTRUCTIONS: This workbook was originally designed to reinforce the information in the most crucial chapter of the book: Chapter 7, Regions and Zones. The extra material in the print version is aimed at helping you assimilate the strategies for Basic HZT discussed in Chapter 9.

If you've got this information, you've got HZT, and at the very least, the simplest level of Hirata treatment, Basic Hirata will be easy to perform.

As well as the diagrams and blank pages for you to colour in, there are worksheets to help you acquire the material. Each task is listed below. When you've completed it, celebrate by ticking it off the list!

- [ ] READ CHAPTER 7

- [ ] READ THE START OF THIS WORKBOOK

- [ ] COMPLETE SECTION 1

- [ ] COMPLETE SECTION 2

- [ ] COMPLETE SECTION 3

- [ ] READ CHAPTERS 5 AND 9

- [ ] COMPLETE SECTION 4

- [ ] COMPLETE SECTION 5

- [ ] REVIEW YOUR ACHIEVEMENTS AND GIVE YOURSELF A REWARD!

- [ ] SHARE A QUESTION, OBSERVATION OR YOUR FAVOURITE DRAWING TO THE ONTAKE GROUP ON FACEBOOK

# LEARNING GOALS

This is a planning tool to get you through Chapter 7 at your own pace. You might do it in an evening, a weekend, a week or a month. Use this planner to help you decide what you want to learn, and when. It's your call!

|  | WEEK 1 | WEEK 2 | WEEK 3 | WEEK 4 |
|---|---|---|---|---|
| MON |  |  |  |  |
| TUES |  |  |  |  |
| WED |  |  |  |  |
| THURS |  |  |  |  |
| FRI |  |  |  |  |

# SECTION ONE

## HOLOGRAPHIC MAPPINGS

**INTRODUCTION**

This section is comprised of two short worksheets, drawing on information in the first part of Chapter 7. You can also refer to Chapter 6. The worksheets are self-explanatory: just answer each question.

# WORKSHEET ONE
### HORIZONTAL ZONES

---

**INSTRUCTIONS**: Answer the worksheet questions below.

"The horizontal zones of the body were always hiding in plain sight in TEAM theory".

QUESTION 1: GIVE ONE EXAMPLE FROM CHAPTER 7 OF A HORIZONTAL LINE OF POINTS THAT JUSTIFIES THIS STATEMENT.

QUESTION 2: GIVE ANOTHER EXAMPLE FROM CHAPTER 7 OF A HORIZONTAL LINE OF POINTS WITH SIMILAR INDICATIONS THAT JUSTIFIES THIS STATEMENT.

QUESTION 3: CAN YOU THINK OF ANY OTHER EXAMPLES, ANYWHERE ELSE IN THE BODY?

# WORKSHEET TWO
## NORMAL AND REVERSE IMAGES

**WHAT IS A NORMAL IMAGE?** PICK THE ONE CORRECT ANSWER.

- ○ It's a holographic representation of the body on a 1:1 scale.

- ○ It's a holographic mapping that goes from medial to lateral.

- ○ It's a holographic mapping that goes from top to bottom.

- ○ It's a holographic mapping that goes from bottom to top.

**WHAT IS A REVERSE IMAGE?** PICK THE ONE CORRECT ANSWER.

- ○ It's a holographic representation of the body on a 1:1 scale but backwards.

- ○ It's a holographic mapping that goes from lateral to medial.

- ○ It's a holographic mapping that goes from top to bottom.

- ○ It's a holographic mapping that goes from bottom to top.

# SECTION TWO

## MEMORISING THE ZONES

**INTRODUCTION**

If you want to practise HZT with confidence, you're going to have to rise to a few challenges, the first of which is to find a way to correlate the number of the zone with its correspondence. If you have a patient with spleen deficiency, you're going to want to apply Ontake to zones 6 and 7 wherever you find reactions. If you see reactions at zone 8, you should be able to interpret that as a sign of kidney deficiency.

This section explores how these same twelve zones repeat in each of the six regions. But first, let's figure out a way to memorise them!

# WORKSHEET THREE
## ZONES AND COLOURS

**GET YOUR COLOURS READY**

**INSTRUCTIONS**: In the left-hand column, continue to list the numbers 1 - 12 with one number on each line. In the right-hand column, list the correlating zone for each number.

Finally, colour in each row in a single colour, or shading style. This will be your key to colouring in the zones and should be kept consistent throughout the workbook.

ZONE NUMBERS

1.

2.

3.

ZONE NAMES

BRONCHI

# MEMORY HOOKS

**INSTRUCTIONS**: On the following blank pages, list zones 1 – 12. Design your own memory hook for each one, or reproduce the ones here but adapted to your own words or visual style. Practise recalling these twelve hooks a few times a day until the numbers and zones are fully integrated and embedded in your mind, and you can call out numbers to zones, or zones to numbers with equal speed.

What mnemonics will you use for zones 4, 5, 6, 7, 11 and 12? Create them and write them down!

**Learning Exercise**

# Bronch-1

Spelt with a '1', not with an 'I'.

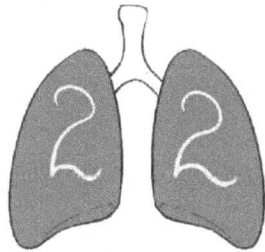

The bronchi split into two lungs.

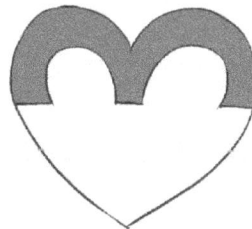

There's a "3" in the heart.

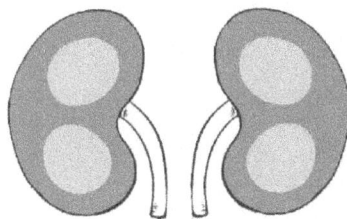

There's an 8 in each kidney.

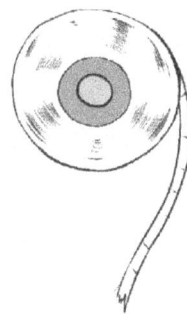

Can we connect toilet rolls with the large intestine?

# Small Intest-10

It's not the best spelling, but it is the best mnemonic!

# JUST DRAW!
## WHAT YOU DRAW, YOU REMEMBER...

# JUST DRAW!
## WHAT YOU DRAW, YOU REMEMBER...

JUST DRAW!
WHAT YOU DRAW, YOU REMEMBER...

# JUST DRAW!
WHAT YOU DRAW, YOU REMEMBER...

# NUMBERING (1)
## SET YOUR STOPWATCH!

**INSTRUCTIONS**: This table lists the zones in alphabetical order. How quickly can you match the zone number with the name? Try doing this out loud. Practise from top to bottom and from bottom to top. Write down your fastest time and the date.

ZONE NAMES                          ZONE NUMBERS

BLADDER

BRONCHI

GALL BLADDER

HEART

KIDNEY

LARGE INTESTINE

LIVER

LUNG

REPRODUCTIVE

SMALL INTESTINE

SPLEEN

STOMACH

Today,_____ my fastest time was_____seconds.

Today,_____ my fastest time was_____seconds.

Today,_____ my fastest time was_____seconds.

# NUMBERING (2)
## BEAT YOUR TIME!

**INSTRUCTIONS**: We're not done yet! Here's a randomised list of numbers from 1 – 12. Once again, try this out loud, at first. How quickly can you match the zone name with the number?  Practise from top to bottom and from bottom to top. Write down your fastest time and the date.

| ZONE NUMBERS | ZONE NAMES |
|---|---|
| 10. | |
| 3. | |
| 6. | |
| 5. | |
| 2. | |
| 11. | |
| 9. | |
| 1. | |
| 12. | |
| 7. | |
| 4. | |
| 8. | |

Today,_____ my fastest time was_____seconds.

Today,_____ my fastest time was_____seconds.

Today,_____ my fastest time was_____seconds.

# SECTION THREE

## INTRODUCTION

By now, you should be very familiar with the twelve zones and able to list them in reverse order while standing on your head and juggling three flaming torches with your feet. This section is even more exciting, focusing on each of the six regions.

There are two processes to complete for each worksheet. One requires your artistic skills and the other guides you to practise in other ways. There's a general checklist on the next page that lists what you should do for each region. In addition to those actions, complete any extra exercises listed on each worksheet.

# ZONE CHECKLIST
WHAT YOU NEED TO DO

**INSTRUCTIONS**: To get the best results from each worksheet, you'll need to do the following:

- [ ] LIST THE LANDMARKS FOR THE REGION

- [ ] DRAW THE LANDMARKS ON EACH REGION IN BOLD

- [ ] COLOUR IN THE ZONES (USE THE SAME COLOUR EACH TIME)

- [ ] LIST ANY OTHER TIPS OR MNEMONICS FROM THE BOOK

- [ ] COMPLETE ANY OTHER INSTRUCTIONS OR EXERCISES

- [ ] REVIEW ONE HOUR LATER (SET AN ALARM)

- [ ] ENJOY THE REST OF THE DAY

- [ ] REVIEW 24 HOURS LATER (SET AN ALARM)

- [ ] PRACTISE ON A FRIEND OR FAMILY MEMBER, ON BOTH THE ANTERIOR AND POSTERIOR SURFACES

# THE ARM REGION
## WORKSHEET FOUR - COLOURING

**INSTRUCTIONS:** Follow the steps of the Zone Checklist on page 18, using the information in Chapter 7 to list the landmarks, mnemonics and zones.

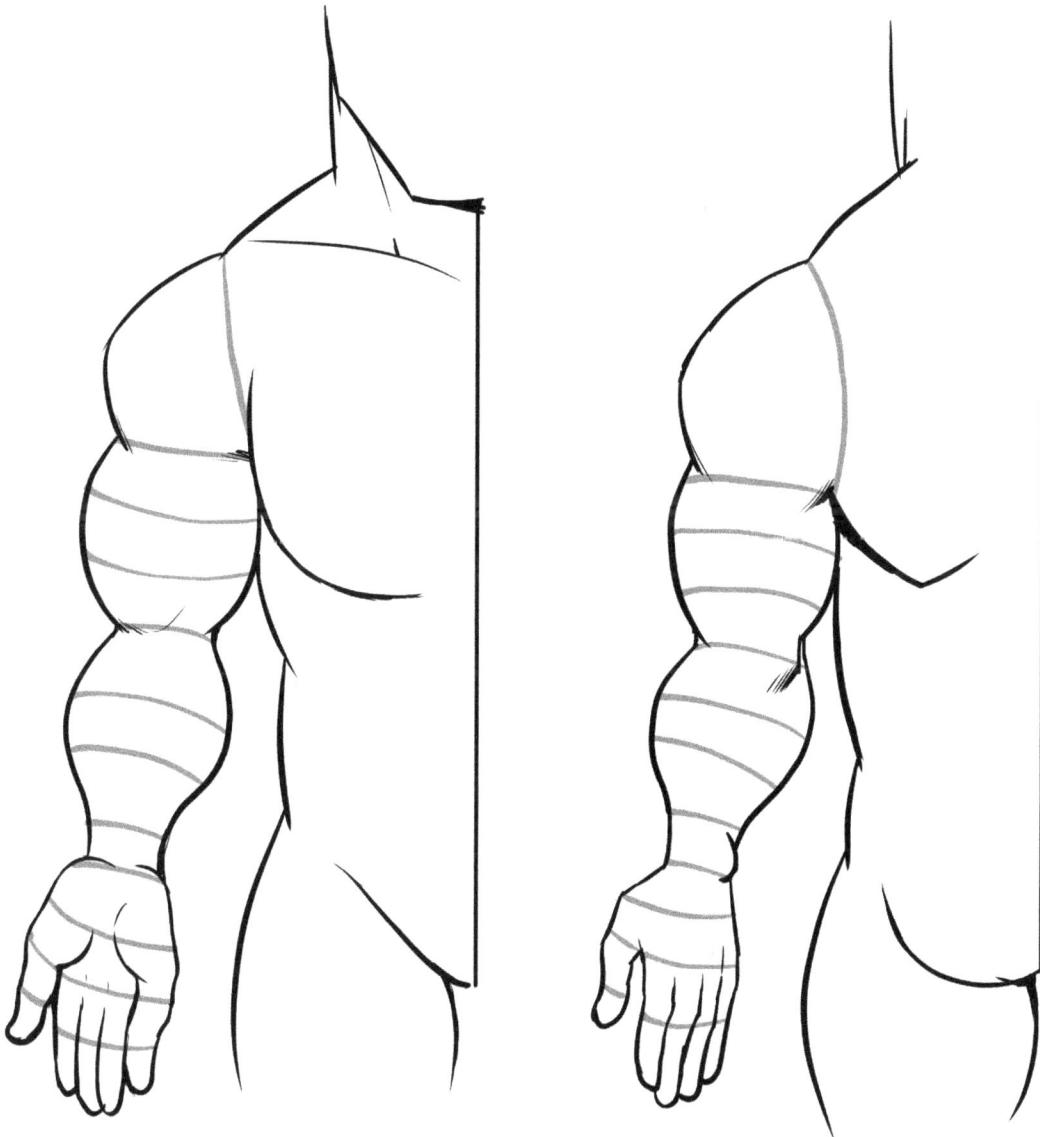

# LEARNING THE ARM
## SOLO PRACTICE

**INSTRUCTIONS:** Using three fingers on one hand as a broad pointing tool, estimate where the arm zones are. Without worrying too much about accuracy, point to where you think zone 1 is on the upper arm. Now point to zone 2. Continue down the arm, until you've touched every zone, all the way down to the fingertips.

Repeat the process, calling out the names of the zones and touching them at the same time.

**THE THUMB:** When considering the thumb, divide the first metacarpal in half at the level of LU 10. This gives you the intersection line of zones 9 and 10. The middle and distal phalanges give you zones 11 and 12.

You can practise this by placing your right hand on your lap, facing up. Put your left thumb on the right LU 9, your left index finger on the right LU 10, your left third finger on the right metacarpophalangeal joint, and your left fourth finger on the right interphalangeal joint. You now can see zones 9, 10, 11, and 12 between your fingers.

Write down your observations in the space below.

# THE LEG REGION
## WORKSHEET FIVE - COLOURING

**INSTRUCTIONS:** Follow the steps of the Zone Checklist on page 18, using the information in Chapter 7 to list the landmarks, mnemonics and zones.

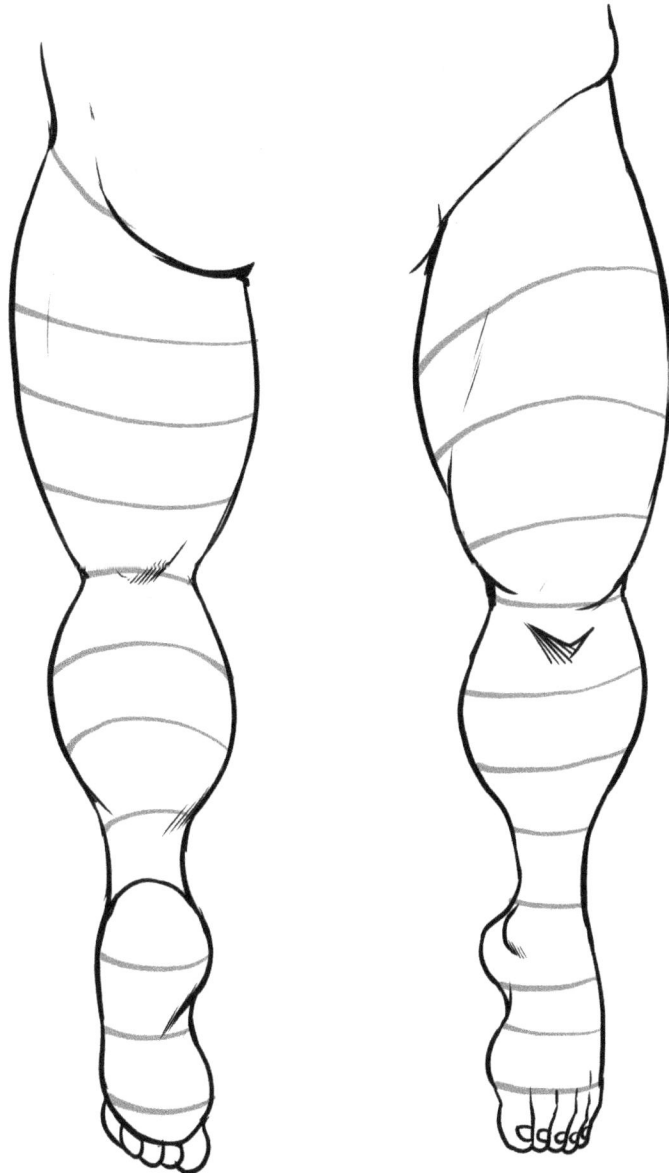

# LEARNING THE LEG
## SOLO PRACTICE

**INSTRUCTIONS**: Using three fingers on one hand as a broad pointing tool, estimate where the leg zones are. Without worrying too much about accuracy, point to where you think zone 1 is on the foot. Now point to zone 2. Carry on all the way up the leg until you're touching your upper thigh.

Repeat the process in both directions, calling out the zone names and touching them simultaneously.

Write down your observations in the space below.

# THE HEAD REGION
## WORKSHEET SIX - COLOURING

**INSTRUCTIONS:** Follow the steps of the Zone Checklist on page 18, using the information in Chapter 7 to list the landmarks, mnemonics and zones.

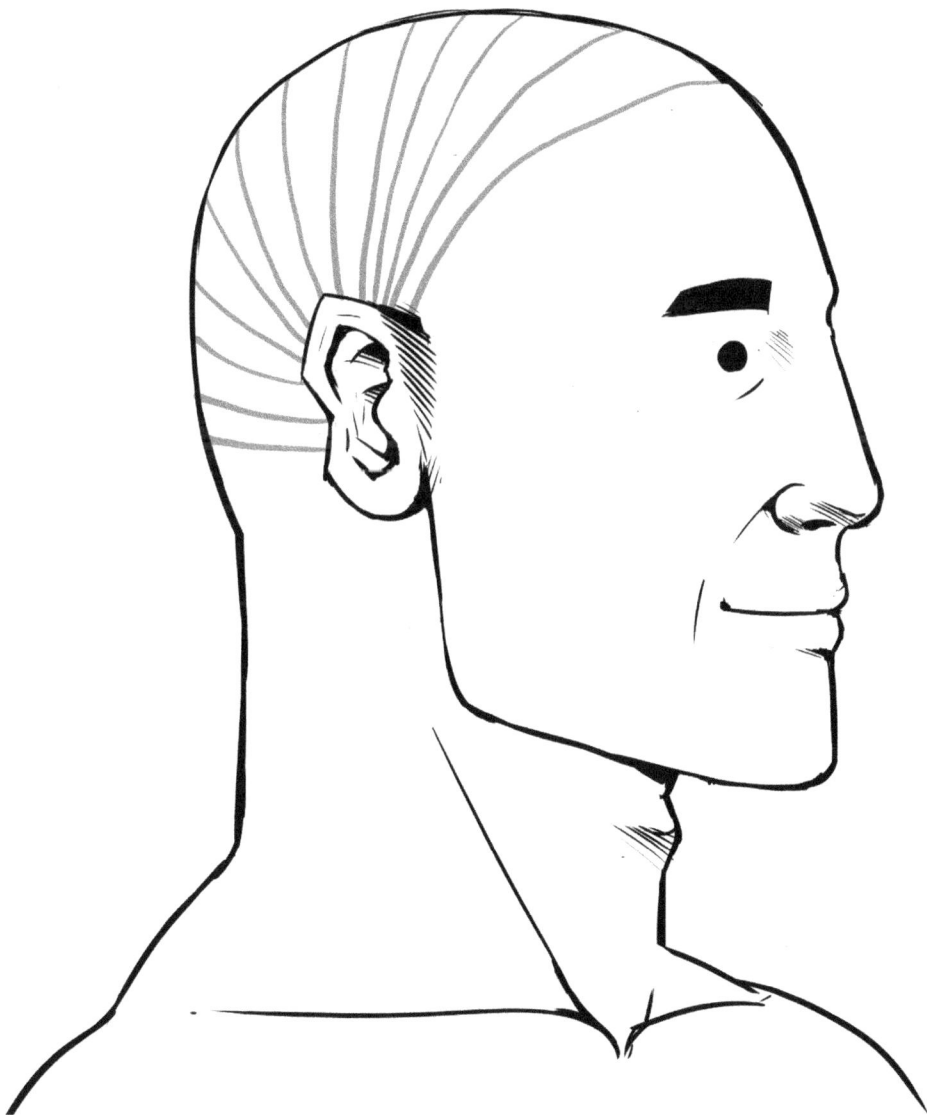

# LEARNING THE HEAD (1)
## SOLO PRACTICE

**INSTRUCTIONS**: Draw an image of a fan with twelve segments in the space below and number the segments from 1 - 12. Write the word "anterior" by the "12" and the word "posterior" by the "1".

Sitting quietly in a chair, imagine a cat perched on your head. Her head is facing behind you, so her tail dangles irritatingly in front of your nose. This means that her zone 1 (bronchi) is posterior, and her reproductive zone 12 is parked nonchalantly on your anterior hairline. Can you draw her?

Write down your observations in the space below.

# LEARNING THE HEAD (2)
## MIRROR MIRROR

**INSTRUCTIONS**: If you consider that this mapping, when viewed from the side, is like a fan, then to practise, you can place an Alice band or a band of cloth over these four landmarks.

You can even use your designer sunglasses as a cool zone location practice tool. Simply push your shades from one of the four landmarks to the next, or use your whole collection.

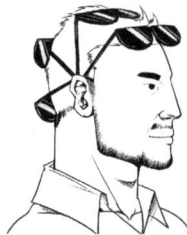

Write down your observations in the space below.

*(Kidnap a family member and practise)*

# THE FACE REGION
## WORKSHEET SEVEN - COLOURING

**INSTRUCTIONS:** Follow the steps of the Zone Checklist on page 18, using the information in Chapter 7 to list the landmarks, mnemonics and zones.

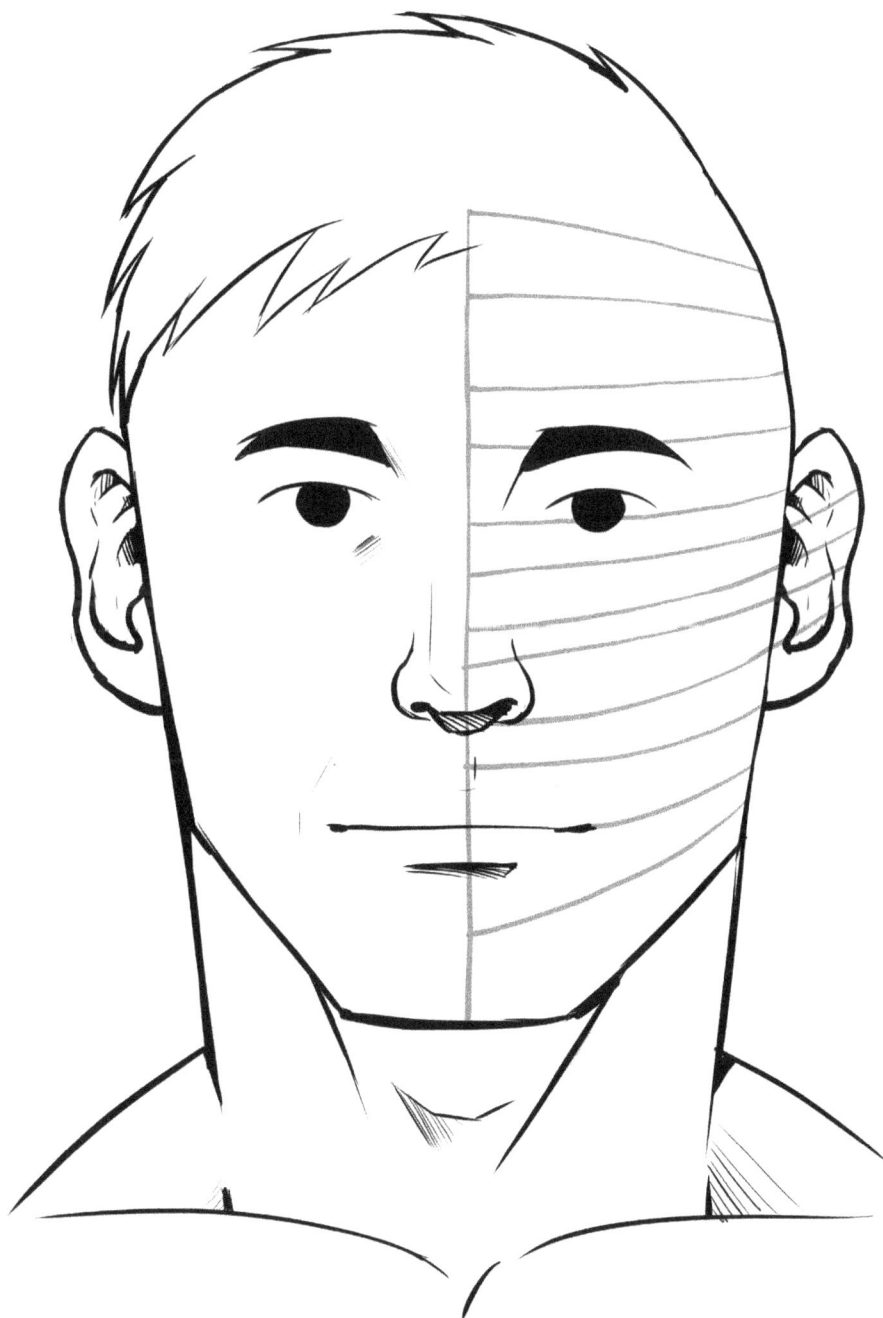

# LEARNING THE FACE
## MIRROR MIRROR

**INSTRUCTIONS**: Stand in front of a mirror and put both index fingers together at the base of your chin. Stroke laterally until they reach the angle of the mandible. This is zone 1. Now place them both at the horizontal groove above the mental protuberance and stroke laterally and posteriorly until you reach the jaw. This is zone 2.

Continue this process up the face until you reach zone 8 and 9 at the outer canthus. You can use two fingers to mark out these zones. When you get to zones 10 – 12, join the middle three fingers of each hand at the midline of your forehead and stroke out with your fingertips until they reach the hairline.

Write down your observations in the space below.

# THE NECK REGION
## WORKSHEET EIGHT - COLOURING

**INSTRUCTIONS:** Follow the steps of the Zone Checklist on page 18, using the information in Chapter 7 to list the landmarks, mnemonics and zones.

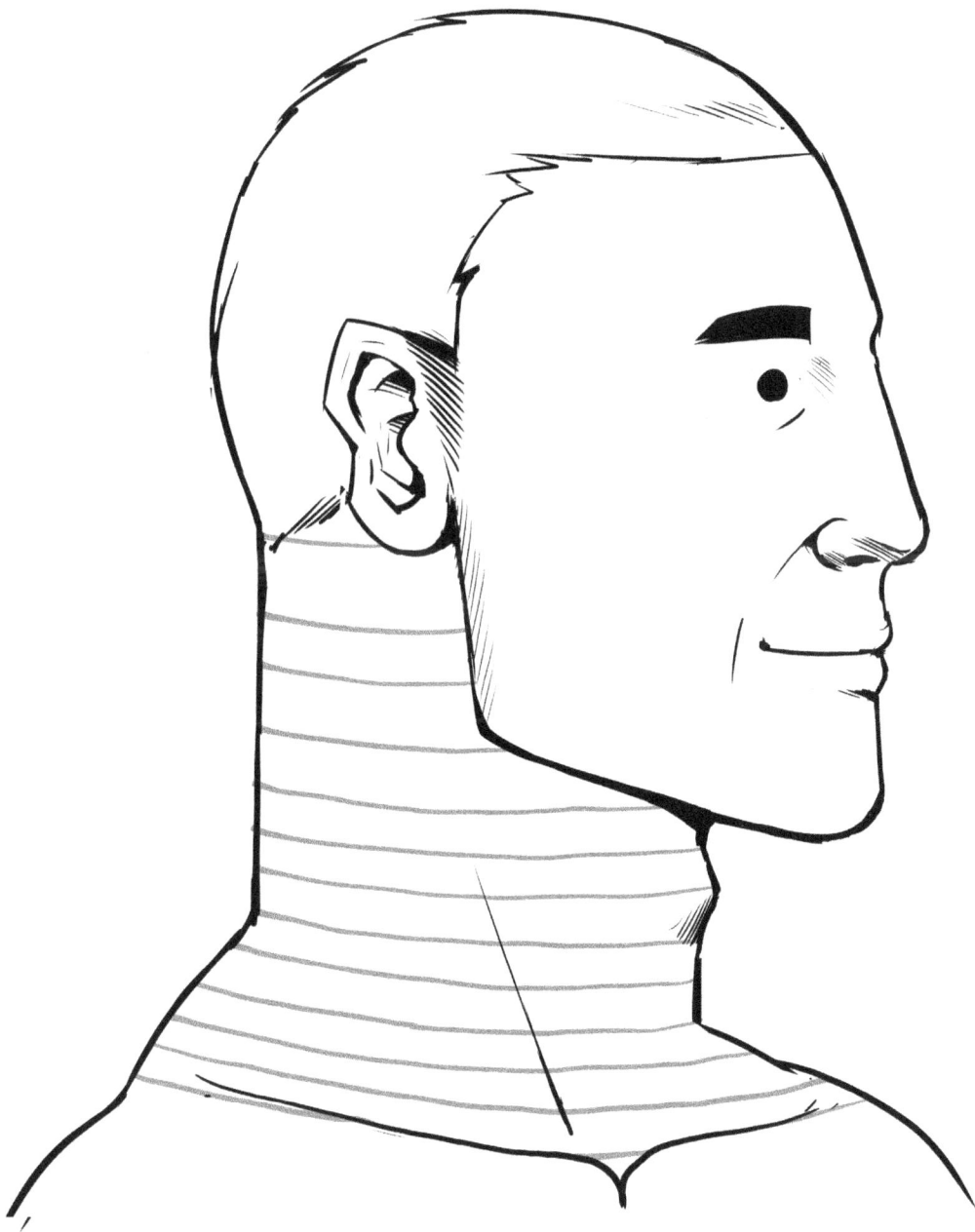

# LEARNING THE NECK
## MIRROR MIRROR

**INSTRUCTIONS**: Standing in front of a mirror, rest your fingers directly on your clavicle on one side. This is zone 1.

Place one finger on each side of ST 9, at the level of the tip of the Adam's apple. Above this level is zone 7; below is zone 6.

Place one finger into the little hollow behind the flap of each ear (just behind the temporomandibular joint). Now move them medially, so they meet at the centre just below the external occipital protuberance. This is the level of zone 12.

Now you have these landmarks, try stroking each zone in-between.

Write down your observations in the space below.

*(Kidnap a family member and practise)*

# THE TORSO REGION
## WORKSHEET NINE - LANDMARKS

**INSTRUCTIONS:** Follow the steps of the Zone Checklist on page 18, using the information in Chapter 7 to list the landmarks, mnemonics and zones.

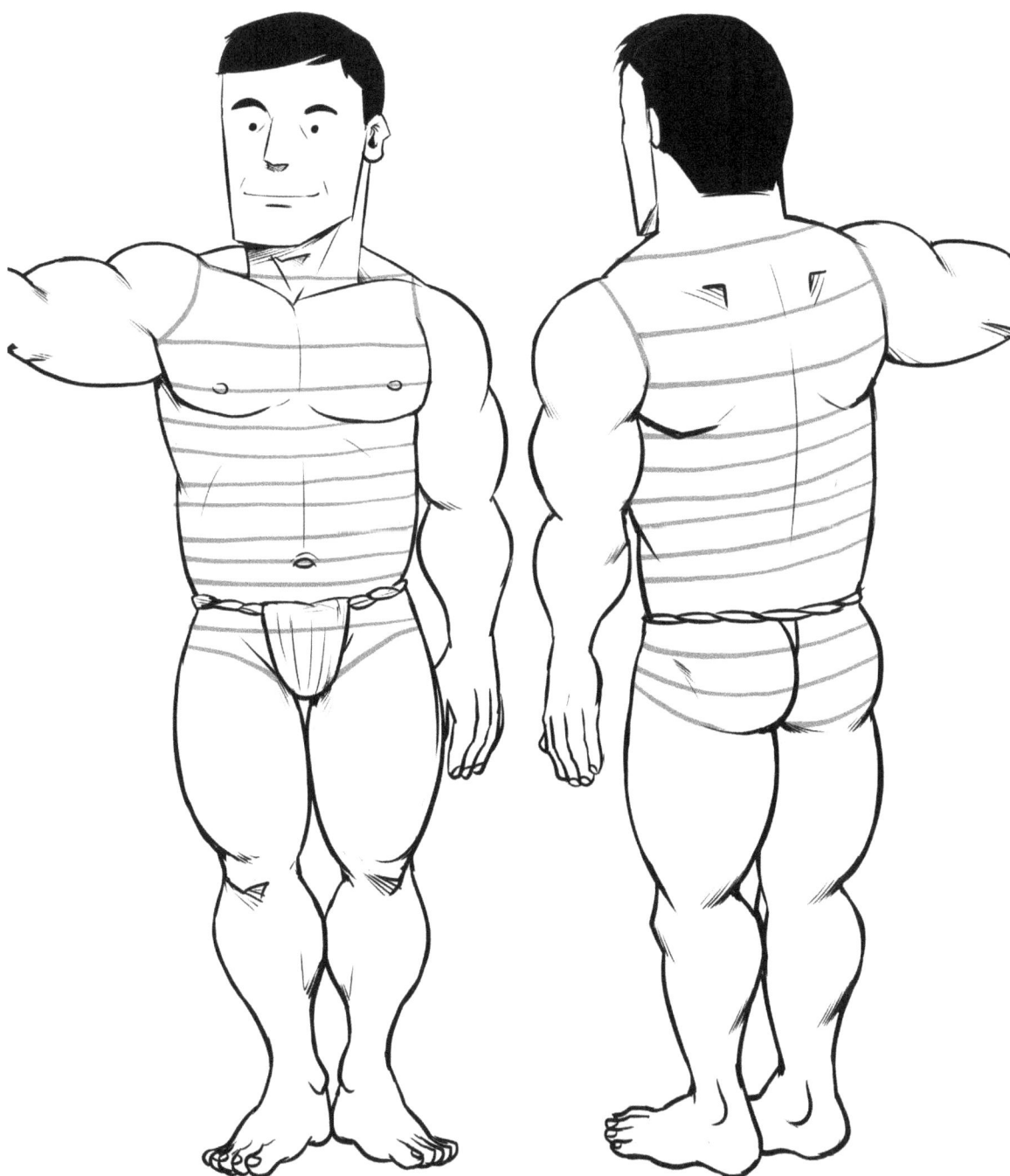

# THE TORSO REGION
## DRAWING FREESTYLE!

**INSTRUCTIONS:** This time without a grid, follow the steps of the Zone Checklist, using the information in Chapter 7 to draw in the zones and landmarks.

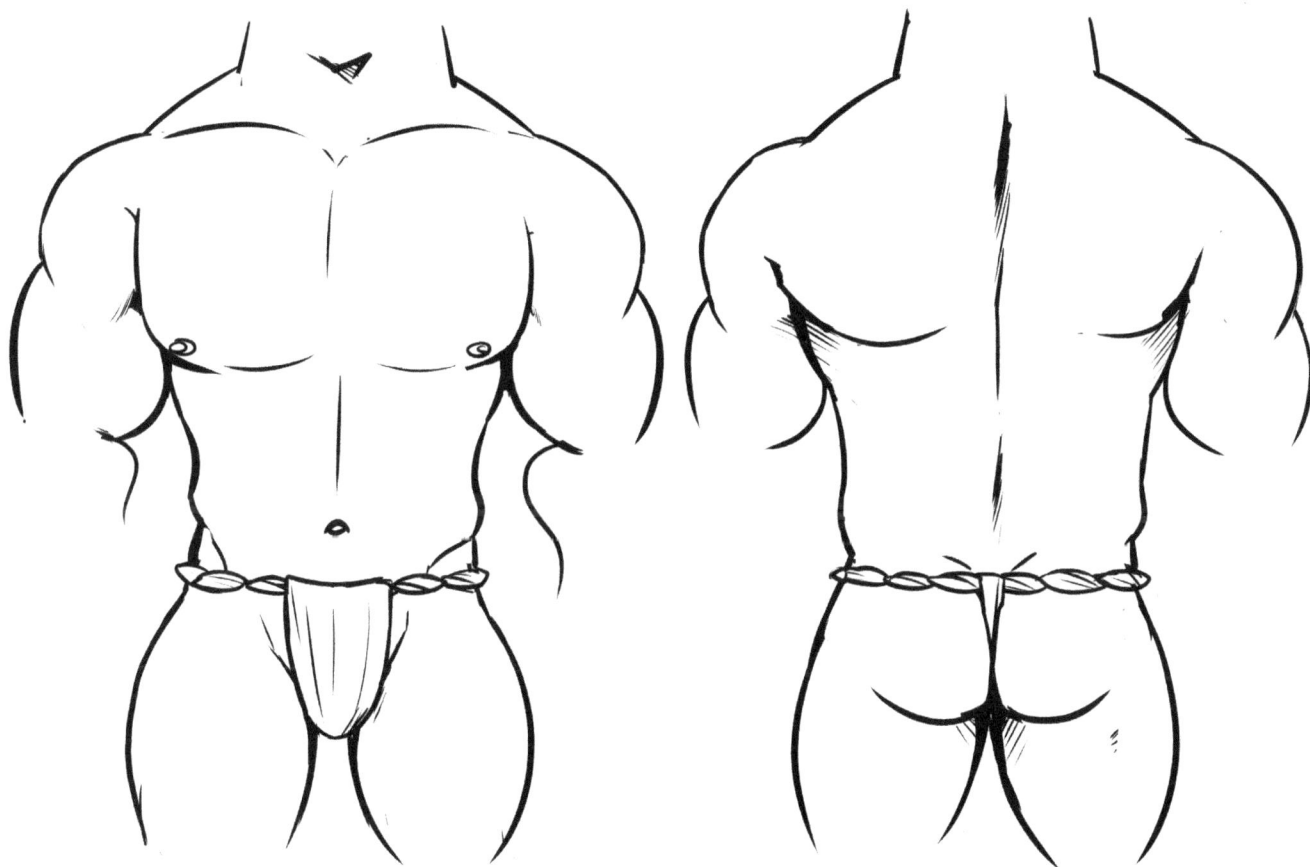

# THE TORSO REGION
PARTNER UP!

**INSTRUCTIONS**: The torso region is the biggest part of the body and probably the hardest to learn, as it's not something you can easily map on yourself.

There are two ways to approach this:

The first is with a partner, mapping the zones out with a marking pen. The second is by simply treating one or two of these areas on your next patient, using the landmarks and related back-*shu* points as starting points.

For example, when you have treated zones 6 and 7 using REN 12 as a landmark a few times, or zones 8 and 9 using the navel, the torso region will start to seem more familiar.

Write down your observations in the space below.

*(Kidnap a family member and practise)*

# SECTION FOUR

## STRATEGIES FOR BASIC HZT

**THE SIMPLEST METHOD OF APPLYING ONTAKE ON THE ZONES**

Now that you've learned the locations of the zones in all six regions, it's time to examine the simplest way to treat them: Basic HZT. The material in this section refers to Chapter 9 and Chapter 5, especially pages 51 - 53.

Basic HZT has the advantage of being easy to teach to your patients, so don't be afraid to share some Ontake and moxa with them, as well as some simple instructions.

# WORKSHEET TEN
## ZONE SELECTION

**INSTRUCTIONS**: Answer the worksheet questions below.

BASED ON THE PRINCIPLES OF ZONE SELECTION FOR AURICULAR THERAPY, WHAT ARE THE THREE CRITERIA FOR ZONE SELECTION FOR HZT?

● Selection according to _____

● Selection according to _____

● Selection according to _____

USING THE TABLE OF DISEASES IN CHAPTER 9, WHY DOES IJTA RECOMMEND ZONES 1, 2 & 3 FOR SHOULDER PAIN? TICK THOSE THAT APPLY.

☐ For anatomical reasons: zones 1, 2 and 3 traverse the shoulders.

☐ For TEAM thinking: the lung channel affects the shoulders.

☐ For correlations with Western medicine: painful shoulders are a classic symptom of flu.

USING YOUR COLOURING CHARTS, TAKE FIVE MINUTES TO REVIEW THE LOCATION OF ZONES 1, 2 & 3 IN ALL SIX REGIONS

WHICH **ONE** OF THE FOLLOWING ZONES IS RECOMMENDED IN THE TABLE FOR HIGH BLOOD PRESSURE? WHY?

☐ Zone 4          ☐ Zone 12

☐ Zone 3          ☐ Zone 8

WHEN YOU ARE TREATING THE TORSO REGION, FOR WHICH OF THE FOLLOWING CONDITIONS SHOULD YOU TREAT ON THE SAME SIDE?

☐ For mild gall bladder or liver dysfunction (treat on the right).

☐ For mild stomach or spleen dysfunction (treat on the left).

☐ Treating directly over an organ.

☐ All of the above.

WHEN IS TREATING ZONES OF THE TORSO REGION ON THE SAME SIDE AS THE PROBLEM CONTRAINDICATED?

☐ When the patient is a woman.

☐ When the patient is a man.

☐ When there is severe inflammation or pain in the organs.

☐ When the patient has mild symptoms.

# WORKSHEET ELEVEN
## ZONE SELECTION

**INSTRUCTIONS**: Answer the worksheet questions below.

WHY DID MANAKA LEAVE PATIENTS ON THEIR OWN WITH
A TICKING METRONOME?

☐ The hypnotic sound helped them drift into sleep.

☐ The clicking sound would keep them awake.

☐ He thought the sound alone could stimulate the channel.

☐ He was quite forgetful.

WHAT POSSIBLE BENEFITS ARE THERE TO TAPPING THE
ZONES USING A METRONOME?

☐ It adds rhythm and predictability to the session.

☐ The ticking sound works isophasally with the rhythmic sensation of heat

☐ The zones might respond isophasally to the meridian frequencies.

☐ All of the above.

**INSTRUCTIONS**: In the left-hand column, continue to list the twelve meridians, as well as the Ren and Du Mai. In the right-hand column, list the frequency for each meridian.

MERIDIAN

MERIDIAN FREQUENCY

1. LUNG

126

2. LARGE INTESTINE

3. STOMACH

4.

5.

6.

7.

8.

9.

10.

11.

12.

13.

14.

**INSTRUCTIONS**: In the left-hand column, continue to list the zone names. This should be easy by now! In the right-hand column, list the hypothetical frequency for each zone.  In most cases, this will match Dr Manaka's meridian frequency. In other words, liver zone and liver channel can both be tapped at 108 bpm.

| ZONE | ZONE FREQUENCY |
| --- | --- |
| 1. BRONCHI | 126 |
| 2. | |
| 3. | |
| 4. | |
| 5. | |
| 6. | |
| 7. | |
| 8. | |
| 9. | |
| 10. | |
| 11. | |
| 12. | |

# WORKSHEET TWELVE
## THE BAMBOO MINI

Unless you have someone to practise on, all these observations may feel like abstractions. The solution is to put the book down and go practise! The best place to start doing Ontake is on the back. It's a broad region, full of different areas with different muscle tone, skin tone, and temperatures. By far, the most important area to consider is the bladder channel, running on either side of the spine.

The Bamboo Mini is a sequence of strokes, working from the top of the shoulders to the sacrum, which is a useful way to close a treatment. Oguri sensei from the IJTA says that treating here "wakes up the immune system". Hirata used a similar protocol for patients with anxiety. This sequence is very relaxing. Before you try it out on a person, try drawing the strokes on the diagram overleaf.

## SEQUENCE
**Tops of the Shoulders**
1. The shoulders are mostly covered by the gall bladder and small intestine channels, which respond to 120 beats per minute. Tap the scapula and trapezius lightly with the mouth of the bamboo (120). As this is a broad area, it can be useful (and soothing) to tap in double time.
2. Roll the same area, focusing on and adapting your depth and strength to the areas of *kyo* and *jitsu* (120).
3. If the top of the trapezius remains stiff, try rolling at 152. Vibrating can be very useful here. If the trapezius still doesn't relax, treat SI 9, 10, and especially SI 11 in the infraspinous fossa (120).

**Back**
4. Tap the bladder channel on either side of the spine (112). Some people find it easier to work from T1 to T7 first and then proceed to the lower points. Others like to connect the whole back in one long sequence. There's no right way, just go with what suits you.
5. Roll lightly on *kyo* areas and firmly on *jitsu* (112). Lean on especially *jitsu* areas for four or eight beats, and then roll afterwards.
6. For urinary, gynaecological, and sacral problems, roll over the sacrum (104). Standing the bamboo on each of the lower Du Mai points for one bar is very relaxing. Stand the bamboo below L2 for one bar, below L3 for another bar, below L4 for another, and continue.

# LEARNING THE BAMBOO MINI

**INSTRUCTIONS**: Using the sequence on the previous page, draw in the areas and lines that you will treat on the model below, as well as the frequencies for each.

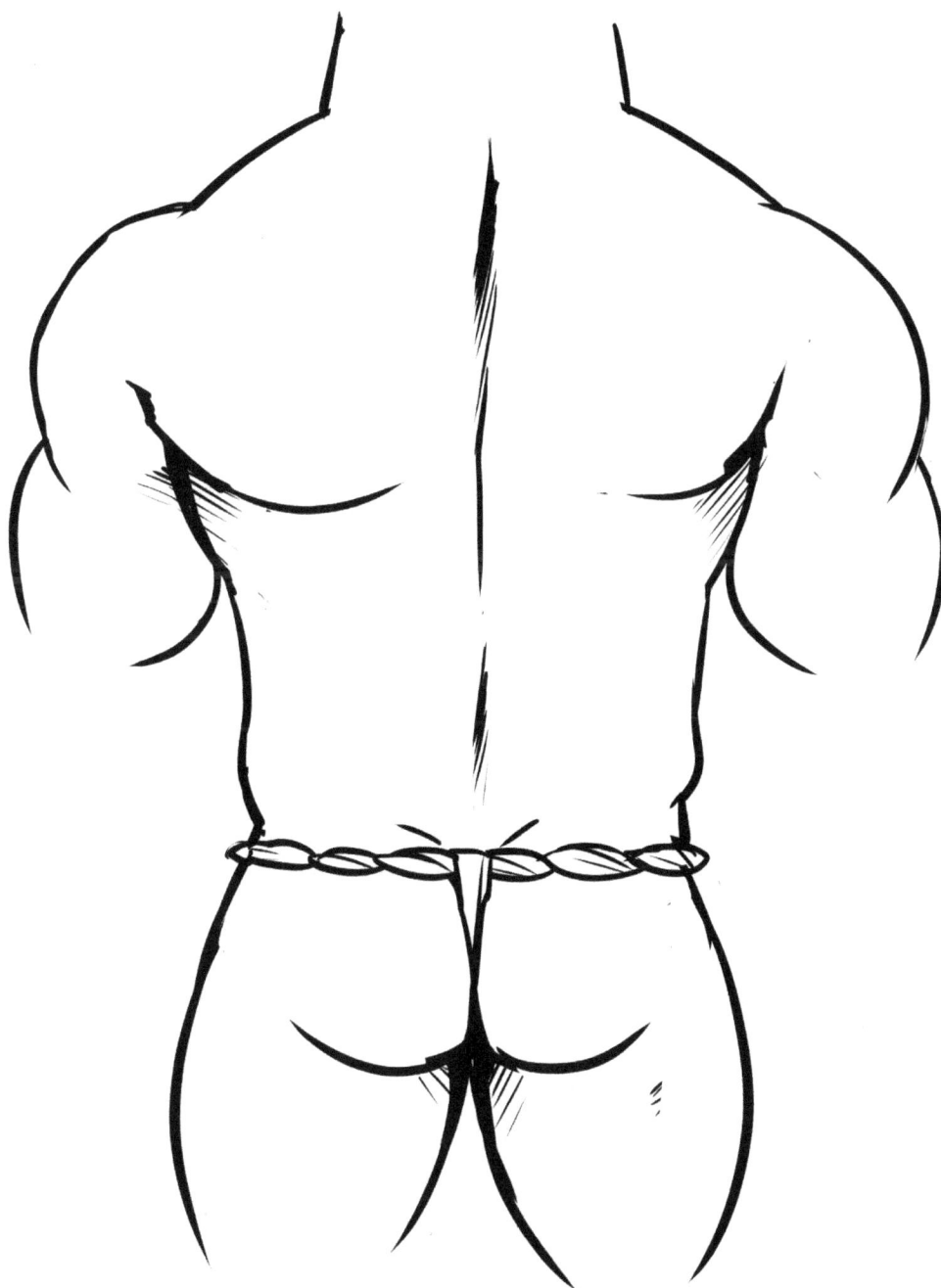

## CELEBRATING YOUR ACHIEVEMENT

Well, you've done it! Hopefully, by now, you can:

List the twelve zones and point to their locations in any of the six regions.

- Set a metronome to the appropriate frequency for a meridian or a zone.
- Select zones according to correlations to Western medicine, TEAM and anatomical location of symptoms.
- Perform the Bamboo Mini, working on either side of the spine to wake up the immune system (and calm the mind).

You should definitely celebrate this achievement by rewarding yourself - you choose! All that remains in this section is a blank page for you to write down questions or observations. For example, you might be unsure if you got some of the answers on the worksheets right.

There's also a list of resources that you can access online. If you've done some artwork that you'd like to share, feel free. The Ontake group on Facebook is a friendly and engaged online community, and we'd love to see what you come up with. And we'll put you straight on your questions.

Your next quest is to figure out how to apply this theory to real people and situations. There are more complex treatment models described in the book that you may also like to adapt, especially when you become more confident in your Basic HZT.  For this, you need to go back to the book and study more!

As time goes on, I'll be devising courses, both online and in-person, so watch out for emails from *The Ontake Method,* which will have news of study opportunities to come.

# QUESTIONS & "AHA!" MOMENTS

This is the place to write down any questions that come or any insights, observations or realisations. Feel free to share any of these with the Ontake community on Facebook.

## FINAL THOUGHTS

First of all, thanks are due to my good friend Reza Gunawan in Jakarta, who read the first draft of the main book and advised me to go more "workshoppy". Thanks also go to Brenda Loew in Seattle, who suggested publishing this extended print version.

Creating all this has been fun! I learnt a lot for myself, not just about conceiving study materials but also about book design and layout. Apparently, diagrams in a colouring book are better printed single-sided! Thank you to Jiet Wong in Malaysia for a two-hour Zoom call picking out all my graphic design "challenges" and many more hours of artistic input, including the front and back covers.

This little side-project has given me great ideas for how to teach this material in the future. I hope it helps you on your Ontake path too.

Of course, studying is an ongoing process that is helped by being in a community. Feel free to join the Ontake group on Facebook, to check out the videos on YouTube and of course, to sign up to my website so you can get Hirata and Ontake news and updates.

*Oran Kivity*

Kaohsiung, Taiwan, 2021

## FEEDBACK

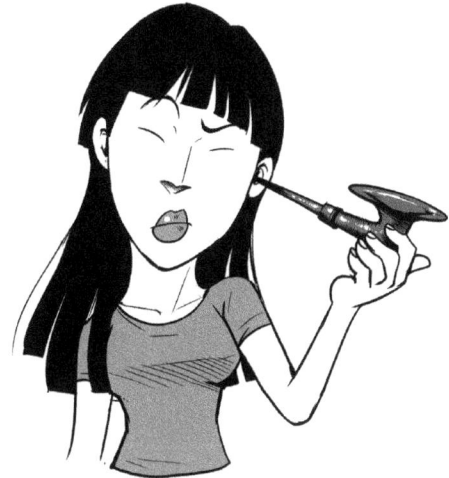

If you've got suggestions to improve this book, please email me (link below). And if you enjoyed it and found it useful, there's no better way to show your appreciation than by leaving a review.

You can do this on Amazon or Goodreads, letting others know what you thought of the main book and, of course, this study book. Thank you!

## ONLINE RESOURCES

Youtube.com/theontakechannel

Facebook.com/groups/ontake/

orankivity.com/shop/

Email: launchteam@orankivity.com

www.ingramcontent.com/pod-product-compliance
Lightning Source LLC
Chambersburg PA
CBHW080901030426
42336CB00016B/2979